AMAZON

A PATIENT'S GUIDE TO LIVING WITH ALZHEIMER'S AND OTHER DEMENTIAS

A GUIDE TO SURVIVAL

By John Caro

PREFACE TO THE PRINT EDITION

Thank you for purchasing this book. It was originally written for Kindle and relies on links to make understanding easier for dementia patients. While it is complete as printed, I strongly suggest you go to the online Kindle store and click on the "Free Reading apps button". You will be taken to a page that offers several choices, click on the "Read instantly in your browser" button to download the Kindle app on your computer. If you have purchased this book, you can download a Free copy for your Kindle. You should download the Kindle App. There are many free books for Kindle, try "ROUGHING IT" by Mark Twain. I laugh every time I read it.

Written in an easy to use eBook form by a dementia patient for other patients, this is a guide to survival in the world of Alzheimer's and other dementias. It tells you what to expect, how to handle the changes, and how to slow the progression of the disease.

2/10/2014

ISBN: **1495224961**

ISBN 13: **978-1495224966**

About This Book

If you bought this book because you are worried about your memory and have not seen a doctor, STOP READING AND MAKE AN APPOINTMENT. There are several conditions that cause problems, like tumors or infections that need prompt treatment.

This book is for those with dementia. I have repeated important information in several places in slightly different ways. This is not a mistake. When you see something that looks familiar, it is important. The guide is to help you through the changes that have occurred and the changes that will occur in the future.

I know you are confused and afraid of what will happen to you. I knew very little when I started this journey and I've had to dig through a lot of misinformation to find the reality behind dementia. No book can cover it all, so this is meant as a guide to start your search. I wish I'd had it when I started.

The advantage of the e-book format is that it uses links. Click on a link and you will be taken to the site. This is far superior to a print book's list of further reading recommendations. You need to be connected to the Internet to use the links here, so I recommend you have your Kindle program on a desktop computer. You can use the free Kindle app on Amazon to download Kindle to any device. A portable device may be lost, but you can always find your desktop. I hope you find this information and the web links useful. The Alzheimer's Association website, is Alzheimer's Disease and Dementia | Alzheimer's Association a good place to start http://www.alz.org/ . You may need to use the Control (CTRL) key when you click on a link. The CTRL key is at the bottom of most keyboards on both the left and right.

Alzheimer's is a slowly spreading deterioration of the brain just as rust is a slow deterioration of steel. I believe Alzheimer's catalyzes Alzheimer's just as rust promotes rust. Iron rusts very fast in salt water but will last for years in fresh water. In the same way, the hormones released by fear and frustration act like salt water on the brain, while the hormones of relaxation greatly slow the progress of Alzheimer's. We are not meant to handle extended stress; it kills our brains. People who are in constant pain for extended periods lose as much as 10 percent of their brain volume. Learning to relax is not just a way to feel better, it is a survival strategy. You are looking for a way to survive; that's why you are reading this book.

I like to use jokes to illustrate my points. Here's one.

There were once two boys hiking in the mountains. They saw a bear, and it began chasing them. The boy in the lead stopped to tie his shoes. The second boy yelled at him, "What are you doing? We'll never outrun the bear!" The first boy finished tying his shoes and said, "I don't care about the bear, I just want to outrun you!"

The moral of this story is don't panic, take your time, and use the links. Your best chance to outrun the bear is to understand and adapt to what is happening. Successful treatments for dementia are very likely to be available in the next few years. Your job is to stay ahead of the bear until then. For more on the adverse effects stress can have on your health, check out this YouTube video from AsapSCIENCE: "Can Stress Actually Kill You?" (https://www.youtube.com/watch?v=vzrjEP5MOT4). The answer is yes it can, but oxytocin the cuddle hormone, reverses it nicely.

Introduction

Twenty years ago, I began having memory problems.

They weren't too bad at first, and I blamed them on stress and lack of sleep. I was a merchant marine and I often worked twenty-hour days, so it made sense that my long hours and demanding job would take their toll on my mental state. However, the problems grew worse. I knew something was wrong when I found an important entry in my log that I could not remember writing. It was in my handwriting and just fifteen minutes old. My brain never formed the memory of writing it.

Over the next few years, I tried to find out what was wrong. I found it impossible to remember names. It became hard to learn new things. I started to hallucinate. I tried going to doctors, but they couldn't seem to find anything wrong with me. I had an ultrasound test to see if I had good blood flow to my brain, and the results were normal. I went to my ship's medical officer and explained my problems. We went through his library and could find only one diagnosis that seemed to fit my symptoms: early-onset Alzheimer's.

I did not know very much about Alzheimer's. I thought there would be some type of treatment I could have, something that would make me better. The medical officer did not want to scare me, so he told me to see my doctor when we returned to San Diego. I saw my doctor, who ran a number of different tests. The doctor was able to determine that the cause of my problems was actually a tumor the size of a grapefruit. They were able to remove the tumor, but my brain had been crushed. I have now been a dementia patient for fifteen years. In that time I have had to deal with doctors both good and bad, along with a drastic loss of income and a string of scam artists who prey on disabled people.

When faced with any type of adversity in life, you have two choices. You can give up and let it roll over you, or you can step up and face the challenge head on with inner strength, faith, and as much humor as you can muster. I chose the latter. I decided that I would not give up. Instead I built a new career caring for people who were in the last part of their lives. I even became a massage therapist with special training in massage for the elderly.

This brings me to the first lesson of this book: stop worrying about your own problems and try to help others with theirs. Volunteer with the Alzheimer's Association or Hospice if you can.

Understand the Disease

One of the things I've learned is that you *cannot give up* if you are diagnosed with dementia or Alzheimer's disease. You are the one who has the power over how you feel and how you deal with the diagnosis. Your attitude will help to guide your family and friends on how they too can handle your diagnosis and the changes that are coming in your life.

It isn't your fault that you can't remember things. You did not do anything to get this disease. It wasn't any lifestyle choice that you made. It's just something that happens to people. Understanding this and knowing that you do not have to hide yourself away and let the disease take over your life is very empowering.

Something else that can help to empower you is knowing more about the disease. Knowing what the disease is and what will happen gives you more power over it. You can pull open the curtains and strip away the frightening mystery of Alzheimer's. The disease is unlike many others that afflict people today. There is no pain, unlike with arthritis, cancer, and other illnesses. Because there is no pain, it is easier to maintain a positive outlook on life. You can look forward to each day as an adventure. Colors become more intense, sounds more interesting. You will be living in the moment in a way that only people with Alzheimer's can. Pay attention—you may be surprised by what you see.

Never Give Up

I've collected books all my life. My favorites are those by authors who write about personal experiences. They may not be the best writers, but they share their experience and that makes their books worthwhile.

I want to share my experience with dementia with you. To get the full meaning of this book, you must use the links. The understanding of dementia is changing daily. The best place to keep up is at the Alzheimer's Association website, http://www.alz.org/ .

One of the things I've found over the years I've spent working with patients is that their outlook affects the progression of the disease. Those who have good humor and a great outlook experience a slow progression. Their zest for life, love, and laughter make a real difference. They are much happier too. On the other hand, those who sink into a depression find that the disease progresses faster.

I believe that it is possible to slow the spread of Alzheimer's. This is a controversial belief. Most books say it can't be slowed. But I have worked with Alzheimer's patients for years and suffer from dementia myself. In my own observations, people who are able to smile and laugh have a much slower progression than people who give in to fear and panic.

I also believe there will be an effective treatment in the next few years. Hang on, it will come. On average, the life expectancy following a diagnosis of Alzheimer's is eight to ten years. However, it can be as much as twenty years. You don't know how long you have, you have so plan on twenty. Who knows what medical advances could be made in that time?

In all my study of dementia, I have never found a book written for patients by a patient. That's why you are now reading this. I wanted to provide information and answers to patients who had questions. Those answers can give you the power you need to take control of your life again.

I hope you find this book helpful.

John Caro

Table of Contents

Chapter 1

The Fear of Alzheimer's

Feeling as though your memory might be slipping is an alarming thing. In fact, when it happens to most people, they want to deny it. They don't want to see the problems that are right in front of them, and they instead pretend the problem doesn't exist, or they blame forgetfulness on stress or lack of sleep. No one wants to feel as though his or her memory or mind is slipping.

In the beginning, the onset of Alzheimer's or dementia is very subtle and goes almost unnoticed. Small things disappear in the beginning, such as birthdays or anniversaries. It's common for people to forget what they deem the little things, and most people see it as no big deal. And in some cases they're right—it isn't a problem. Everyone experiences trouble remembering things from time to time. But the forgetfulness and memory troubles may go much deeper. If you are forgetting more things now than you did six months ago, it's time to tell your doctor.

If your memory problems are being caused by an illness, it is important to know as early as possible. You could be worrying about nothing, or you could have a tumor. When you know you may be dealing with dementia or Alzheimer's disease, you can confront the issue and deal with the changes that will be come into your life. It's always better to face a problem head on than to ignore it and let it worsen. In this book, I'll show you how to do that.

Many Feel the Same Fears

Alzheimer's has become the new bogeyman. People fear it more than cancer or heart disease.

Twenty years ago, AIDS was the bogeyman. It was not well understood, and there was no effective treatment. AIDS was a death sentence: nobody lived more than ten years, and treatment seemed impossible. People who were HIV positive lost hope and often killed themselves. My brother's best friend was one of them. But then effective treatments were found, and much faster than anyone thought possible. HIV is now a treatable condition, like diabetes or heart disease. It is no longer a death sentence and therefore no longer the bogeyman.

I believe Alzheimer's is in the same situation now that HIV was twenty years ago. A cure, or, at least an effective treatment, will be found soon.

A recent study from the MetLife Foundation, which put out an Alzheimer's survey conducted by Harris Interactive, showed that more people in the United States feared getting Alzheimer's disease than feared having diabetes, stroke, or heart disease. (You can learn more about this by visiting the links at the end of this chapter.) The study went on to say that eight out of ten people felt it was important to prepare for the disease, but more than 80 percent of those people had done nothing about it. They were afraid, but it seems as though they wanted to ignore the possibility of a problem, just as most people do. It's unfortunate but true. Most people know very little about Alzheimer's and have no idea what to expect, or even what they should look for when it comes to the signs and symptoms. But ignoring the problem is not a solution.

You Are Not Alone

Even though dealing with a diagnosis of dementia or Alzheimer's might be a frightening time for you, it's important to know you are not alone. Approximately six million people in the United States have Alzheimer's. These people are dealing with the same fears and problems you are, and that means there is help. You can find the information, support, and guidance you need to understand and handle these changes in your life. Fear tends to feed on itself. I'm going to show you what I did to break the downward spiral of fear.

This book is here to help you understand all you can about dementia and Alzheimer's, and to provide you with links and resources to help you even further. Your life might be changing, but it's still your life and you can take control.

It's time to do some learning. Use these links to find the latest information.

Chapter 2

Basics of Alzheimer's and Dementia

People often use the terms dementia and Alzheimer's disease interchangeably. However, there is a big a difference. There are many different types of dementia, some of which can be treated. It is very important to find a doctor who understands the differences and gives you the right treatment. The wrong treatment can make your illness worse or even lead to death.

A bit of information on Alzheimer's, as well as the history and discovery of it, arms you with more knowledge. Remember, the more knowledge you have about Alzheimer's, the more power you have over it. Besides, it is an interesting disease.

What Is Dementia?

Dementia is a term that refers to a set of symptoms; it is not a disease itself. Dementia is the loss of cognitive function, and it ranges in severity. In the beginning, the symptoms are generally mild. As dementia progresses, symptoms become worse, as is often the case with other types of medical issues. Some of the symptoms of dementia include:

- Trouble finding the right words
- Trouble remembering recent events or activities
- Trouble planning tasks
- Trouble doing various tasks
- Depression
- Less attention to personal care and grooming
- Problems recognizing places and face

We'll go over more of the symptoms in detail in the next chapter.

Unlike dementia, Alzheimer's is an *actual disease*. It is the most common cause of dementia. However, it's not the only cause. In the next chapter, we will look at some of the ways to determine whether you are really suffering from Alzheimer's or if it is another form of dementia, such as vascular dementia, which causes a change to the blood supply in the brain.

In addition to the two main reasons for dementia—Alzheimer's and vascular dementia—other things can cause these symptoms as well, including:

- Side effects from medication
- Brain tumors
- Brain infections
- Vitamin B12 deficiency
- Blood clots in the brain
- Lewy bodies, abnormal aggregates of protein that can cause dementia
- Parkinson's disease
- Frontotemporal lobar degeneration
- Creutzfeldt–Jakob disease
- Alcoholic dementia
- Huntington's disease
- An excess of toxins like mercury or lead

What Is Alzheimer's Disease? Use this link What Is Alzheimer's Disease?

YouTube - https://www.youtube.com/watch?v=9Wv9jrk-gXc

As mentioned, Alzheimer's is a disease, whereas dementia is the term for the symptoms that make up the disease. Dementia is the catchall term for the symptoms you are suffering from.

Alzheimer's is a progressive brain disease that has no cure yet. This can be frightening to discover—I know it scared me. Don't forget, many other diseases are incurable, like diabetes or heart disease. They are treatable, though. A person with diabetes can live a normal life, and so can someone with heart trouble. Keep your spirits high and keep your faith. Have a sense of humor and look for the positive things in your life. Each moment is a gift that you can accept with joy or reject with fear. It is your choice.

In most patients, the symptoms and the disease do not develop until age sixty to sixty-five. Treatment and a positive outlook can slow the progression of Alzheimer's. While there is currently no cure or way to reverse the disease, I believe there will be soon.

Receiving a diagnosis of Alzheimer's is frightening. It is like standing on the edge of a cliff. Nobody wants to die; nobody wants to have an incurable disease. But even though there might not be a cure for Alzheimer's yet, that does not mean you have to shut down your life. You are alive, and where there is life there is hope.

Instead of worrying about the lack of a cure, look for a cure. Spend some time on the Internet. Find a good clinical trial and enroll. Think of yourself as a soldier in the fight. Or you could just give up. It's your choice.

You have a lot of time. It is much better to look for the elements of fun and humor in life. It makes the time you have much happier, and it will slow the disease.

How Does Alzheimer's Affect Your Brain?

Your brain takes in information through your senses and processes it to control your body and your environment. It has to create an electrochemical analog of your environment to function. Think of it as a mirror of reality. Most of us think that what we are experiencing is reality; the mirror is very good, after all. But the truth is that you are aware of what your brain is creating, not what is really around you. For instance, you have no sensory organ that detects the electric fields in your home, even though those fields are strong in places. Some people think the fields have an effect on your cells and so try to avoid them. You can find these fields with an AM radio. Put it between stations and turn up the volume, then move it around your computer. You will find a louder hiss on one side than the other. That is the power supply. You can go around your house and find the strongest fields if you like. It is a good idea to avoid them. They may cause problems with your health and thinking. This is just an example of the difference between reality and your perception of reality.

It is important to remember that Alzheimer's will change your perception of reality, but it cannot change reality itself. When I worked on boats, we often had new hires who became very seasick. They lost touch with reality and could not tell which way was up or down. I found that I could cure most of them by telling them to remember that the bottom of the ocean was solid and not very far beneath our ship. They only had to change their thinking to stop the panic. Despite what their eyes were telling them, gravity does not come from different directions, it comes from the center of the earth. This is what we mean by getting your sea legs—sailors are connected to the center of the earth, not the rolling boat. So it is with Alzheimer's: you have to realize that your perception of reality will change, but reality itself is still the same. Find your center now; it will keep you from panicking later.

Alzheimer's is a slow destroyer of brain cells. It starts in the hippocampus, the part of the brain that forms new memories. That is why it is considered a disease of memory. It continues on to the part of the brain that handles speech, then to the part that handles reasoning, then to the emotional center, then to the sensory center (sometimes causing hallucinations), then to the back of the brain where the oldest memories are stored. At the most advanced stage, balance and breathing are affected, and you pass away in your sleep. The progression from one part of your brain to another is what defines this disease. It spreads from the center to the front, over the top, and down the back of your brain. This is roughly the reverse order in which your brain developed. You will become more childlike as the disease progresses.

Here is a riddle. A pond is being covered with water lilies. Each day, the lilies double in number. If the pond is ten acres and is completely covered with water lilies after one hundred days, on what day was the pond only half covered? You don't need a complex equation to solve the problem—the answer is ninety-nine days. Remember, the lilies double every day, so the day before the pond was completely full, it was half full. Similarly, Alzheimer's moves through the brain from cell to cell, and one cell affects several other cells. You can slow this spread by reducing your number of fear hormones, such as cortisol, that kill brain cells. You can also increase the number of protective hormones, like those produced by laughter, that slow the spread of

Alzheimer's. You can't stop the disease completely, but slowing the spread is a very good thing, especially in the earliest stages.

Consider this sequence: 2, 4, 8, 16, 32, 64, 128. Now consider this one: 2, 8, 32, 128. In the first, the numbers double; in the second, the numbers quadruple, increasing at twice the speed of the first sequence. Now suppose someone finds a way to stop the spread of Alzheimer's three years from now. This is very possible, given the present stage of research. Where do you want to be in three years? At 16, a stage at which you are still able to function almost as well as you did before, or at 128, a stage at which you are greatly impaired and unable to function?

I know this sounds grim, but did you honestly expect to live forever? Imagine if you had been diagnosed with cancer and had only six months to live. I have cared for several cancer patients. Most were surprised by the degree of pain at the end. They would have given anything to have a single day without pain. With Alzheimer's, however, you have years ahead of you. You can choose to live in fear and frustration, or you can choose to take each moment as a gift. Think about it. You don't have unlimited time—no one does—but you can choose how you spend it. Spend it wisely. I'll tell you what I did in the next few chapters.

Keeping Positive

Your brain classifies everything as Bad, as in "Oh no, it's a bear, run!," or Good, as in "Relax, we got away." Once your brain has decided if something is good or bad, it knows which of your two peripheral nervous systems to activate. If it is a bad thing, your brain will activate the sympathetic nervous system, preparing you for fight or flight by shunting blood from your internal organs to your muscles. Healing and digestion stop. Your breathing and heart rate go up as adrenaline pours into your body. You are ready for escape. Running for your life uses up fear hormones. That's why exercise helps you relax. When you are afraid, it helps to take a walk to calm down.

If your brain has identified something as good, it will activate the parasympathetic nervous system, which prepares you to rest and recuperate. Digestion and healing resume as soothing hormones pour back into your system.

The best way to fight your dementia is to walk, then relax and realize the bear is a long way away. There is no reason to run from it. When you finish your walk, use a cool, wet cloth to wash your face. This activates your diving reflex, slowing your heart and causing the capillaries in your skin to contract, forcing blood to your internal organs. You can use deep, slow breathing to massage your heart, which moves up and down with your diaphragm and releases calming hormones when it is moved.

Your brain acts as a mirror of the things around you. Try this. Take a mirror and smile at yourself. You may not feel like it, but fake it for five minutes. What started as a fake will become real and you will feel better.

Joke with the people around you. You will all have more fun. Laughter is real medicine, it lets your body and soul heal, and it feels good too.

One of the best things I've done is to stop watching the news. My stress level dropped considerably and I find I can pay more attention to the reality of my life. This does not mean you're ignoring the world, you're just choosing what you expose yourself to. The purpose of most news programs is to make you watch the commercials anyway. Television programmers call it delivering eyeballs. The most effective way to deliver eyeballs is to say something scary like “Up next, is something in your refrigerator about to kill you? Stay tuned for more.” Then, once they have your full attention, they move to commercials trying to sell you soap, a new car, yucky diet food, hamburgers, and then that car again. In the first two seconds of each commercial, there is a hook to make you keep watching. It may be a bell or buzzer, or a question like “Gee, Sally Mae, how do I get my laundry as clean as yours?” My favorite is simply “Hey, look at this!” My point is that the “news” is not really about what happened, it's just something to keep you watching the commercials. Try giving up FOX or MSNBC or CNN for a week and replace it with soft music. I am listening to meditation music as I write this.

You will find yourself much happier if you joke with the people around you. They will joke back and you will both have fun. Laughing activates your rest-and-relax system. It is healing medicine.

You have years ahead of you. Enjoy each moment. Find something that works for you. Staying as positive and happy as possible is the best way to slow your disease. It also improves quality of life, for you as well as your family. Instead of wallowing in despair, find new reasons to smile and laugh. You'll find that your family will follow suit and adopt your positive attitude. This helps your life once again take on a brighter and broader scope.

In the end, having a great quality of life and spending happy times with your loved ones are really the things that matter. Relax and let yourself enjoy life.

What Is Early-Onset Alzheimer's?

As you might guess from the name, early-onset Alzheimer's occurs when a person develops the disease at a younger-than-normal age. Estimates are that about 5 percent of those who have Alzheimer's disease are younger than sixty-five, and they are considered to have early onset. Those with early-onset Alzheimer's are generally in their fifties. In my case, I was diagnosed at forty-eight. However, there are cases of people being diagnosed even earlier, as young as their thirties. This is very rare, though.

Those who develop early-onset Alzheimer's may have other members of their family, such as parents or grandparents, who developed the disease early. Families that have a tendency to develop Alzheimer's early should watch for symptoms of the disease.

Get Your Family Ready

If you developed Alzheimer's early, it is important to talk with your family so that they too can watch for symptoms that might affect them when they hit their thirties, forties, or fifties. Knowing what might be coming will allow you to take steps to care for the problem. In fact, this is true whether early-onset Alzheimer's runs in the family or not. Being prepared is always a good idea.

If early-onset Alzheimer's runs in your family, all of your relatives should buy long-term care insurance *before* they are tested for the disease. Most insurance, including Medicare, does not cover nursing home care. A positive test for Alzheimer's may make it difficult to purchase long-term care insurance.

See the links below to learn about the many things you can do to prolong your useful time.

Links:

AboutAlzOrg: "What Is Alzheimer's Disease?" (YouTube video) - https://www.youtube.com/watch?v=9Wv9jrk-gXc

National Institute on Aging: About Alzheimer's Disease: Alzheimer's Basics http://www.nia.nih.gov/alzheimers/topics/alzheimers-basics

Mayo Clinic: Alzheimer's blog http://www.mayoclinic.com/health/alzheimers-disease-and-dementia/AZ00053

National Institute on Aging: "Inside the Brain: Unraveling the Mystery of Alzheimer's Disease" (video) http://www.nia.nih.gov/alzheimers/alzheimers-disease-video

Mayo Clinic: Early-Onset Alzheimer's http://www.mayoclinic.com/health/alzheimers/AZ00009

PBS: William Thies, Ph.D., Chief Medical and Scientific Officer, Alzheimer's Association, discusses the benefits of early detection (video) http://www.pbs.org/wttw/retirementrevolution/2009/08/06/william-thies-ph-d-chief-medical-and-scientific-officer-alzheimer%E2%80%99s-association/

Chapter 3

Is It Really Alzheimer's Disease?

Your memory loss might be the onset of Alzheimer's, or it might be a simple matter of being forgetful occasionally. The following are some of the early signs and symptoms, which can help you have a better idea of whether you might be suffering from Alzheimer's. However, you should always visit your doctor to make sure that you are getting the right diagnosis and the proper help for your condition, whatever it might be. In the next chapter, we'll go over how to choose a quality doctor, and what to expect when you go in for your visits.

As promised in the last chapter, the following is a deeper look at some of the signs and symptoms that generally affect those who have Alzheimer's disease. These are the types of things that you will need to expect and prepare for as the disease progresses. Yes, they are scary, but you can take control of them.

Memory Loss Disrupting Your Normal Routine

Perhaps the most known and recognized symptom of dementia and Alzheimer's disease is memory loss. You might forget information about something that happened quite recently. For example, you may not remember what you had for dinner, or you may not remember writing a letter to a friend. You might forget the plots of your favorite movies or whether you've seen the latest episode of that television show you love. Of course, the remedy is to watch them again. After all, you liked them the first time, right? In addition, sufferers will often forget dates of special events, such as birthdays. You might find that you increasingly need to ask people to repeat information. I have found that people get mad when I have to ask them the third time. I tell them that my hearing is bad so they don't get upset.

You will also find that you need to rely on your family quite a bit more when it comes to remembering different things. Other memory aids, such as notes around the house and on the refrigerator, might help you to remember too. Just be careful not to overdo it. Two or three notes help; twenty or thirty will just add to the confusion. I use a large calendar to help me keep track of daily happenings. There is plenty of room to write and it lets me stay organized. No more forgotten birthdays!

Forgetfulness is a nuisance, but it can also be dangerous. I almost burned down my house when I forgot to turn off the stove. I now only use cooking devices with timers. When I forget about my food, the microwave or toaster oven turns itself off. You can never be sure when you will have a blank spot in your memory when you have dementia. I recommend you switch to automatic cooking *before* you have a fire.

You may forget to do important things, such as taking your medication. Alternatively, you might believe you've forgotten to take your meds, and you could take a double dose. If you take medication daily or weekly, it is important to have a pillbox with the days labeled on it. Only put in a dosage that's right for a single day. I use a weekly pillbox with a.m. and p.m. sections. If I forget to take a dose, I leave it in and take the dose for the correct day. That way I can tell if I have taken my dose by looking at the box. It helps me avoid taking a double dose. Make sure you find a way that works for you to take your meds properly. This is very important.

As the disease progresses, so does the severity of the memory loss. It's generally a gradual slide, so you can do certain things to help prepare for this. The trick for dealing with memory loss is to replace functions you lose with things in your environment. For instance, if you can't remember your phone number, write it on your phone and on a card in your wallet. You are probably going to have times when you can't remember things followed by times that you can; even worse, you may give the wrong phone number and not know it. Reading it off your handset will give you the confidence to use your phone again.

Look for help from family and friends, home medical care, and more of those reminders. Some patients today are using audio, video, and written reminders for various things. You may want to try these as well. I will go into detail about this in a later chapter.

Greater Difficulties Completing Regular Tasks

You will find that all of the normal things you once did are a bit more difficult now. You might have trouble remembering the way to work or to the grocery store. You might forget the layout of the grocery store, too. This makes navigating more difficult, time consuming, and even dangerous. When you are lost, don't panic. If you are driving, pull over and ask for directions. If you are walking, take a break. Rest will often restore your memory.

Keep Safe

When you have trouble knowing where you are going when you are walking or driving, it could be dangerous to go out alone, and it is very dangerous to drive. As much as you might not like it, giving up the keys could be one of the best things you can do. You will find this hard, but do it anyway. Operating a car is one of those skills that still work when you can't think, but driving is much more than operating a car. I suggest you sell your car so you don't forget and drive it. Use the money for taxi fare. You will avoid a lot of trouble.

Walking is a different matter. It is very good exercise and should be part of your life as long as possible. When I go outside for a walk, I simply follow the same road until I'm tired and then turn around and return to my home without having to remember turns.

Difficulty with Problem Solving and Following Directions

Another thing you will experience is greater difficulty solving problems. Whenever you have to do something, even if it is something familiar, you may have trouble. For example, you might have issues reading and following directions from a map. You might have difficulty with simple mathematical problems, which was never an issue before. One of the reasons for this is that you are having a difficult time concentrating. It will be difficult to focus for long periods. When you find that this is happening and you recognize the problem, take your time. Slow down with the problem, and if you feel your concentration flagging, quit for a while and return to it later.

Your brain has to construct a picture in your head to match the real world. It uses both electrical energy and neurotransmitters to do this. With dementia, the brain makes fewer neurotransmitters than normal. When they are used up, you feel tired and can't think. Some of the dementia drugs block the uptake of these neurotransmitters and give you a more normal supply. I take 10 mg of Aricept twice a day to improve my thinking, but I still have to take long breaks to let my brain recharge.

Visual Issues

You might find you have some issues with your vision as well. Many patients have some trouble when it comes to judging distance. This can lead to problems with balance, and will likely cause problems with driving. When you can't tell how far away something is on the road, an accident is inevitable. Things may seem perfectly normal to you until you pull out in front of a truck.

Other visual issues could come into play as well. For example, you may have trouble when it comes to determining colors. This can cause difficulty with driving, choosing clothing, and even some work-related issues. But a lot of people are diagnosed early now and still are able to work for several years. I know a woman who is in her eighties and still runs a large seafood restaurant even though she has an impaired memory. She has always treated her employees like family and they take care of her like a mother. The restaurant grosses about three thousand dollars a day. Dementia did not mean the end of her life, and it does not have to mean the end of yours, either.

Time and Place Confusion

Many people with Alzheimer's have trouble when it comes to understanding time. They may not always recognize where they are or when they are. They might not know how they came to be at a certain place. They might even mistake certain people for other people in their life. I sometimes have this problem. I tell myself that I am *here* and the time is *now*. This helps me to not panic. I hope that if I ever mistake someone for someone else, they will understand, but if they don't, too bad—I won't remember the incident long anyway.

There is a movie on Netflix called *Memento* that shows the effect of not having a short-term memory. When you watch it, note that the hero is quite intelligent, but his memory only lasts a few seconds. Also pay attention to the part about subconscious learning in persons with memory loss. One scene shows a test to expose fraud in a person faking memory loss. The person is told there is a test of dexterity in which they pick up objects and place them in the correct order. One of the objects is electrified and gives a painful shock when touched. The test is repeated several times. A person with genuine short-term memory loss will learn to avoid the object. They won't know why, but they don't want to touch it. A person faking it for insurance will keep picking it up. They are willing to put up with a little discomfort to get a pension. This demonstrates that there is more than one place in the brain that stores memories. You can store behaviors (like putting your keys in the same place) deep in your brain in order to replace being to remember where you left them. Dementia does not mean stupidity.

Verbal Communication Issues

Are you feeling as though you have difficulty getting your point across? Are you having trouble knowing which words to choose? I know I do. This short book has taken more than two years to write. This symptom is another frustrating and embarrassing one. You may forget the words for familiar items you have all around the house. It can make talking with people at work difficult too. I have found that it is best to say, "I'm sorry, I've lost my words" when this happens.

This symptom can make it difficult to follow conversations as well. If someone asks you to do something, you might not understand the instructions. You might need them repeated a few times before you can do what is asked. Asking for written instructions is better than trying to remember what was said. I carry a pocket-size notebook for writing things down. I just say I'm hard of hearing and hand over the book. It saves a lot of embarrassment.

Losing Things

Anyone can misplace things. It happens all the time. But when you have dementia, it gets much worse. You are going to get a lot of practice searching for things. Here is my secret for finding lost items. First, look where you think it is. Not there? Ask someone if they have seen it. No luck? Look in the places it should not be. For instance, I often put my wallet in the freezer. Still no luck? By now you are probably upset. Take a break and reset your attitude. It isn't your fault, it is just the disease. Your frustration will keep you from finding your item. It's like standing on a trap door. You can't open it until you step off. The sooner you learn to relax, the less trouble you will have remembering where you left your stuff.

There will be times when you just can't find what you are looking for. That's when you have to say, "I give up looking." This happens to me about ten times a day. Often my item is found right after I do this, though sometimes it isn't. That's life.

At first you will want to blame someone else for taking your stuff. It will make you mad, and you will focus on them instead of your search. When this happens, take a break and let yourself relax. If you must blame something, blame your disease, because it really is to blame.

Bad Judgment

Bad judgment can plague those who have dementia and Alzheimer's, often because they simply do not remember making a decision.

It's unfortunate, but there are scammers who try to take advantage of those who are disabled. They are very good at locating us. Your best protection is to simply not talk to them. I recommend you screen your calls with caller ID. Some will still get through, though, and you should hang up as soon as someone says "you've won" or mentions money. If you do win something, you will be notified by registered mail. That's the law.

Nobody calls you to give you a medical device either, not ever. Medicare has a lifetime limit on what they will pay, and when it is reached you pay for your own care. Medical devices can be amazingly expensive. A simple glucose meter that costs twenty-five dollars at your drugstore may be billed at five hundred dollars by a phone-order company. Of course, a scammer will tell you that you will pay nothing because your insurance covers it. As soon as you realize they are trying to sell you something, say, "I never do any business over the phone. Please don't call me again. I'm hanging up now." It's OK to interrupt the spiel. Most will keep trying to talk while you are hanging up. Don't worry about hurting their feelings—this is a total stranger who is trying to cheat you. Don't listen, just hang up.

You may also get investment advice in the mail. None of it is worth your time, much less your money. If you have money to invest, buy a fund that tracks the market, or better yet, look into an annuity that pays you a set amount each month. This is not the time to take chances.

Speaking of chances, you should avoid gambling. You can become more susceptible to thinking you are about to win than a normal person. All of the slots in the world now use computer chips made by International Gaming Technologies, which has a patent on an electronic random number generator that can be controlled from a central location. In other words, the odds can be changed while you are sitting at the machine. When you press the play button, a number is selected and the computer is told whether you win or lose and by how much. The computer then plays an entertaining show that is designed to make you want to play again. If you want to go to a casino for the entertainment, take only what you can afford to lose and leave your ATM and credit cards at home.

Choose a trusted member of your family, or an attorney, to help take care of your finances and affairs. This way you will not be the one in charge of all of your money, and the chance of your being on the receiving end of a con is much lower. It is vital that you choose someone you trust to help you with any financial or real-estate affairs that might arise. Money often becomes a problem in the last stages of Alzheimer's, and you want to be able to trust someone to handle these issues as best they can.

Personal Care

Personal care tasks will become more difficult. You will need more time to brush your teeth and shower, but don't let that stop you. Nothing drives people away like bad breath and body odor.

Mood Changes

Something else that you and your family members may notice as the Alzheimer's progresses is that your mood can change, sometimes very abruptly. Instead of feeling happy, patients will sometimes feel anxious or afraid. They might also become suspicious and even angry. This is partly due to the culmination of the confusion they feel over some of their other symptoms, or it can be caused by the deterioration of the emotional centers of the brain. This can be very dangerous. If you feel yourself becoming angry, try to exit the situation, either by leaving the room or changing the subject. Do your best not to yell at anyone. With Alzheimer's, yelling leads to fighting and fighting leads to legal problems. Direct your anger at the disease, because that is the real problem.

Depression and Isolation

All of these symptoms can cause depression to set in. I mentioned earlier that depression can be very dangerous, but it bears repeating because it is so important. When you feel depressed, you will try to withdraw from your normal life. You will not want to visit with family and friends, and you no longer enjoy life. You become mired in depression and feel bad for yourself because of your symptoms. You believe you can't enjoy the things you once did, and it causes you to withdraw from normal life. If you can't shake the depression, ask your doctor for help. Depression will speed up the progression of Alzheimer's.

Feeling sorry for yourself is normal—we have all done it. It is also a complete waste of time. There is a sign in my favorite nursing home: "Don't cry because it's over, smile because it happened." You have been blessed with a long life and now you are being blessed with a long, gentle ending. Be thankful for the blessing.

Rely on your friends and family, on the things you've always loved, to help bring you out of your depression. Become more active with your family. Take advantage of the great times you have. Make use of your humor and your faith to make the most of your life. Make your peace with the world. You have plenty of time.

Where Do You Fall?

Are you still not sure if you have Alzheimer's? It is true that people forget a few more things as they age, but you are reading this because you are worried.

Getting older will often mean that you will suffer from one or more of these issues, not necessarily because of Alzheimer's, but simply because that's the aging process. We've all spent time trying to remember where we put our keys or what date it is. We all make bad decisions occasionally, and most people forget to pay a bill once in a while. These things happen, even to younger people. As we age, the problems may become a bit more frequent. However, if these problems are chronic and they are worsening, it can be a sign of dementia and possibly Alzheimer's disease. Don't panic; you just need to do what comes next.

What Next?

Whenever you are suffering from these symptoms, whether they seem severe to you or not, you should visit a good doctor. While there are no definitive tests for Alzheimer's, a good doctor can perform a number of different tests that will narrow down your problem.

Alzheimer's is usually diagnosed by eliminating other possible problems. Some of the other problems are much worse than Alzheimer's and need immediate treatment. Alzheimer's does not usually cause headaches, for example, but tumors and infections do. If you are having severe headaches, go to the emergency room. A few weeks after I was told I might have early-onset Alzheimer's, I began to have huge headaches. It turned out I had a brain tumor. My neurosurgeon told me I was only a few weeks from death. If you are having headaches, you may not have time to wait for an appointment.

Headaches can be caused by a number of things, many of them essentially benign, but why take a chance by waiting to be seen? Having your symptom(s) assessed at the ER can save valuable time and avoid prolonged worry.

Alzheimer's is frustrating and embarrassing, but it is not usually painful. If you are having memory problems and are waiting for an appointment, and then have a sudden headache, go to a doctor right away. In this rare case you may have to be treated immediately. On the positive side, many tumors can be removed and you will have a big improvement in your symptoms. We will go over all of that in the next chapter, when we learn more about doctors and what to expect.

Links:

The Alzheimer's Association: Know the 10 Signs -
https://www.alz.org/alzheimers_disease_know_the_10_signs.asp

Health.com: 25 Signs and Symptoms of Alzheimer's Disease
http://www.health.com/health/gallery/0,,20416288,00.html

Chapter 4

Preparing for Your Doctor's Appointment: What to Expect

When you find your signs and symptoms are pointing toward Alzheimer's disease, you should get in touch with a doctor for more information as soon as you can. However, it is important to make sure you are working with a doctor or doctors who can really help you with your condition. It is important to put in a bit of effort to find someone truly qualified. Here are some tips that will help you.

Getting the Right Doctor

Do you know what they call the person who graduated last in his class at medical school? They call that person "Doctor," of course. You probably don't want a person who is barely qualified as a doctor to treat you! Here are some of the things you need to look for when choosing your doctor.

Someone Who Listens

Your doctor should listen to what you say. He or she needs to listen to how you feel, to your symptoms, and to your fears and questions. The most dangerous person in medicine is the very intelligent doctor who is wrong in his or her diagnosis and who won't listen to you.

Whether you are going in for dementia issues and questions or for any other medical reason, it's vital to have a doctor who actually listens and does not automatically believe his or her diagnosis is correct simply because they have a book somewhere that says they *might* be right.

If the doctor does not have time to listen to you, then you do not have time for that doctor. Find someone new.

Someone Who Lets You Know What's Happening

The doctor should explain your diagnosis, as well as what it means for you and what changes you can expect in your life. These are the experts in the field, and they've seen patients who have gone through things similar to you. The doctor should take the time and have the compassion to explain everything that is going to happen. He or she should explain any tests that might be given, along with any treatments that might be tried.

Your doctor should also be honest with you about these treatments. Even though there are a number of different treatments now in use, it is important to remember there is no cure for Alzheimer's disease—yet.

Someone Who Sets Treatment Targets

Having a doctor who knows how to set treatment targets and goals is important as well. When you have a target, it is easier to gauge where you are in the treatment process and how you are doing. In turn, this lets the doctor adjust your goals and targets as he or she sees fit.

Someone Who Reviews the Meds

Every doctor you see should look to see what medications you are taking. This includes prescription meds and any supplements or vitamins you might take. It is important to make sure you provide the info about those supplements. This ensures that the doctor will not prescribe something that could interfere with the meds you are taking already.

Someone Who Has a Good Reputation

Look up some reviews of the doctor to see what type of reputation he or she has in the field. If the reviews are all negative, and they say the doctor does not provide adequate treatment, or that the doctor does not seem to care about the outcome for patients, eliminate that doctor from your list. You want to choose a healthcare provider who has glowing reviews and testimonials from appreciative patients. A good doctor, or team of doctors, really can make all the difference in the world when you are facing something as new and as frightening as dementia and Alzheimer's disease.

Someone Who Helps to Arrange a Caregiver

The doctor likely knows caregivers who can help you and may have staff who can help train members of your family to provide the care you need too. Your spouse is probably best, followed by children or grandchildren. Whomever you choose, make sure it's someone you like and get along with well. Most of the time it is best to have family members help with caregiving, but this is not always possible.

Finding Homecare Service

Another option is a homecare service. Chances are your doctor may know some good options. You can ask for some recommendations, but always take the time to vet the provider, just as you did with the doctor.

If you hire a homecare service, make sure they won't change your caregiver without warning. Also, make sure the caregivers are allowed to lift more than twenty-five pounds and can help in the toilet. I once worked for a company whose insurance would not allow those things.

Another option is to run an ad for a certified nursing assistant (CNA). Expect to pay twelve dollars or more an hour. This is still less expensive than a homecare service.

Make sure you check references and run a criminal background check on *anyone* you hire. You need to know and trust the person you are hiring. It is rare, but some criminals do seek out the disabled. It is in your best interest to check the criminal record of anyone you have in your home.

At first it is a good idea to hire someone for at least a few hours a week to give your primary caregiver a break. Your care team can expand as needed over time. All teams are different, just as all Alzheimer's patients are different. The important thing is that you feel as comfortable as possible with the team you build.

What Happens After Choosing a Doctor?

Now that you have your doctor, it is time to set up your first appointment. You want to do this as soon as you can in order to get the help you need as quickly as possible.

During the initial consultation, the doctor may give you some tests. It is important to remember there are no specific tests to indicate whether you have Alzheimer's or not. The doctor will make his or her determination based on your symptoms. They can generally tell whether you have dementia and whether you are exhibiting Alzheimer's. It is important, therefore, that you are honest with the doctor with all of the questions he or she might ask.

Even though you will not receive a specific "Alzheimer's test," there are a number of other types of tests to help differentiate between Alzheimer's and memory loss associated with age or other types of dementia. The following are tests that your doctor might consider giving you while determining your diagnosis.

Neuropsychological Tests

To determine the extent of your memory problems, your doctor may recommend you see a specialist in neuropsychological testing. These tests determine where your memory issues fall in comparison with other people your age. This provides a benchmark of where you are, and the results will help the doctor determine whether you are likely suffering from the early stages of Alzheimer's disease. The doctor will also have a better idea of your current mental and memory capacity, a useful baseline for the future.

Lab Tests

Blood tests will look for other things, such as a vitamin deficiency, that could be causing your confusion and memory loss. In the case of vitamin deficiency, the doctor will prescribe vitamins to see if it helps improve your memory and cognitive function.

Physical and Neurological Tests

These tests are some of the first the doctor will give you when you go in for your appointment. In fact, he or she may give you these tests on your first or your second visit. They include testing of your balance and coordination, vision and hearing, reflexes, and strength. These tests can help indicate problems you might be facing.

Brain Imaging

With today's advanced medical technology, it is possible to scan the brain and produce images that could indicate changes in mental function. These scans do not detect Alzheimer's disease, but they can detect quite a few different anomalies that could be causing issues in your cognition. For example, they can detect tumors, brain trauma, and more. My MRI showed a tumor the size of a grapefruit. The neurosurgeon told me I would die without surgery—in less than a month. That MRI saved my life.

The Technology and Tests Are Getting Better

Imaging techniques are getting better each year. Soon they may be able to detect some of the anomalies that could be indicative of Alzheimer's disease. These technologies are new, but Alzheimer's treatment is changing fast and you want the best care you can get.

Referrals

Your doctor will likely be able to provide you with some of the preliminary tests to help determine the level of your memory loss. However, he or she will also need to send you to a specialist at some point, particularly for the advanced tests. Some of the different types of specialists you may have to see include:

- Neurologists
- Psychiatrists or psychologists
- Geriatricians

No one likes going to doctor after doctor, but it's essential during this stage. You want to go to the *best* specialists in your area so you can be sure about your diagnosis.

The Benefits of Early Diagnosis

When you begin having memory issues, it's important to quell your fears and visit your doctor as soon as possible. The sooner you are able to get into the doctor's office the better. Early detection is important and conveys a number of benefits, so get into the doctor's office soon.

With early detection, you can start some of the Alzheimer's treatments early, which can give you the maximum benefits. By starting treatments early, you will retain your independence longer. This will give you more time to plan for your future too. You will have more control over your care and living options, and you can take care of financial and legal matters early. With the right plan and the right team in place for when you need it, you and your family can rest easy.

A good doctor will know a good lawyer who specializes in elder law. It's very important that you ask about getting a consultation. You need current advice about the law for your area. It changes very often. I would avoid those "senior retirement seminars," as they are just sales presentations. Be careful of advisors who tell you—usually for a fee—how to hide your assets in order to qualify for Medicaid. You can find yourself in a lot of trouble at a time when you can't think. Pay for the lawyer, it will be worth it.

Having this level of control is something many people do not have because they wait too long to see the doctor and receive their diagnosis. Once again, it is fear that keeps people away from the doctor. But by now you know you do not have to let that fear control you. The greater your knowledge and the earlier you detect this disease, the more power you have. You can be the one who dictates how things progress with your life, and your attitude can make everything easier on you and your family.

What Are the Current Types of Treatments for Alzheimer's Disease?

While there is no cure for Alzheimer's, some helpful treatments are available, and they may be worth trying. I will cover the most common and successful types of treatments in

Chapter 8.

Don't forget to use these links!

Links:
The Alzheimer's Association:Choosing Care Providers
http://www.alz.org/care/alzheimers-dementia-screening-providers.asp

Mayo Clinic: Alzheimer's Disease: Tests and Diagnosis
http://www.mayoclinic.org/diseases-conditions/alzheimers-disease/expert-answers/alzheimers-test/faq-20057850

Chapter 5

Handling Your Diagnosis and Dealing with the Changes

When you first receive your diagnosis, chances are you don't really know what to think. Look at it this way: yesterday you knew you had problems remembering things, but you didn't know why. I remember working out ways of faking it. Now you know the reason. You can relax because it is not your fault. You are not lazy. You are not stupid. You have a disease and now you can treat it. Remember that you have a lot of years left to live. In that time you will live to see better treatment and maybe even a cure.

Start changing your environment to help you function as long as possible. The idea is to replace functions you lose with something else that does the job, like using a pocket notebook to help you remember, or training yourself to put your keys in the same place so you don't lose them.

In these times, your best option is to turn to your loved ones, your humor, and your faith. These things can help carry you through even the darkest of times. Having something to believe in, things to do, and people in your life to love will make a huge difference. You are the one who will determine how you handle the disease, and you can turn the negatives into positive experience. Basically you chose whether you are happy or sad, and why would you choose to be sad?

I've already mentioned that maintaining a positive outlook can make a real difference in your quality of life. It really does help, and even though the first few days after receiving the diagnosis can be terrifying, you will be able to adjust to all of these changes and to conquer your fears. Others have done this and *so can you.*

I have avoided mentioning God and religious belief so as not to offend anyone. However, in my experience caring for dying patients, I have found that people of faith do much better than those who have nothing to believe in. It makes no difference what they believe, only that their belief is strong. Atheists can also have strong central beliefs, but people who are unsure of what they believe have a much harder time.

Decide what you believe in and build your life around it. It takes time, but it's worth it. Remember the Serenity Prayer:

God, grant me the serenity to accept the things I cannot change
The courage to change the things I can
And the wisdom to know the difference

Adjust to the Change

Your life is changing. There is no getting around that. You need to make changes to your environment and your thinking now, while you still can. This means you will need to have some time to adjust to those changes. Different people may take different amounts of time to make this adjustment, so don't feel as though you are floundering if you can't get used to the idea of having Alzheimer's disease after a couple of days. Many patients need to take longer to wrap their head around the diagnosis and to accept it. That's perfectly fine. It is normal, in fact.

Take the amount of time you need to come to terms with your diagnosis, but make sure you are actually trying to come to terms with it! You may have several days where you feel better, and then you might start to feel overwhelmed again. This too is normal. *Take the time you need.*

Too many people will fall into despair and depression during this time. If those feelings of depression are slipping over you, it is possible to avoid or reduce them by doing things you enjoy and being with people you love. They can help support you in this time. If you cannot shake the depression, ask your doctor for help. He or she can suggest treatments that will make it easier for you.

Many people think about suicide after they have been diagnosed with a terminal illness. This is normal, but if you really think that you should kill yourself, read *Final Exit* by Derek Humphry first. You can find it on amazon or E-bay. Suicide affects everyone around you. Read his book before you decide. You have plenty of time and you may decide it would be a mistake.

Get Support

You can find people to help you through this time. Your friends and family are a natural place to start. However, you do have other options that can add to your overall support.

Your doctor will have some names of local groups of people who are dealing with Alzheimer's disease. If not, you should find another doctor. You can look online for some great support groups as well. Start with ALZConnected, the online support group from the Alzheimer's Association. https://www.alzconnected.org/default.aspx

The right support makes all of the difference. Make sure you consider all of the different types of support you need too, including:

- Emotional support
- Day-to-day support
- Household and financial chores
- Financial support

Make Your Plans

Now that you know the different types of support you need, it's important to start making actual preparations for it. You will need to think about how you want your healthcare covered and what you want to happen to your finances. During this time, it is important to speak with your family about the things that are important to you and how you want to proceed with various areas of your life as the Alzheimer's becomes more advanced.

During this stage, it is vital that you choose family members whom you trust implicitly. They will be making your decisions for you when you can't do it on your own, so it's important to entrust the right people with this responsibility.

Preparing for Care

One of the areas I touched on earlier was preparing for physical healthcare and daily care. I can't stress enough just how important it is to find providers who have the skills and the compassion to do the job. Long before you need to rely on the healthcare providers, you should look into finding the best ones. Then when the time comes, they can step in and help. Make sure that you arrange all of the financial matters of your healthcare early too.

In the next chapter, I'll discuss all of the different stages of Alzheimer's disease.

In the earliest of the stages, you will still be able to retain a very independent lifestyle. You will not need to have constant care. As the disease progresses, though, the time will come for your care providers, and often a professional healthcare team, to take over. You will have to let them do so. Don't let it bother you when they tell you what to do. You are going to be living through a reverse childhood and they have to protect you, just as parents protect their children.

The Right Healthcare Provider

Just as you spent time looking for the right doctors, you need to have the right healthcare team ready to provide round-the-clock service and help. Your family members will be able to take care of quite a few different things for you, but eventually they will need help too. You need to make sure your family has quality assistance. Make sure you have your family help you look for a provider. Here are some of the things you should look for with in a healthcare provider:

Experience

How long has the company been in business? How much experience do the nurses, nurse assistants, and other healthcare providers have? Try to choose a facility that can guarantee you will have someone with plenty of experience to help you and your family.

Reviews

Always look up reviews of the company to see what other patients and families have said about them. If the reviewers say negative things about the employees' levels of care and compassion, do not choose that provider. It pays to take the time to search for a truly compassionate team that has your best interests at heart.

Background Checks

The company that provides you with the CNAs and healthcare assistants should conduct background checks on all of their employees. If they do not, you can request your own background check for criminal activity, or you can simply move on and find another provider.

Look for References

Always get at least three references. If possible, call or e-mail people who used the provider so you can ask about their experiences. You can ask the family some questions you might not feel comfortable asking the provider, and you can be sure you are getting the real information. This helps keep you from choosing the wrong provider, as many can "put on a good show" and be very charming while they are trying to get your business. The references will let you know how the provider works with patients after the checks are cashed.

In-Person Visit

Always schedule an in-person visit with the provider and the people who will be working with you. It's better to get a sense of the people who will offer the care, and it can ensure that everyone's personalities work well together.

Care Plans

What types of care plans does the provider offer? Do the patient and family members have input into the care plans? The provider should always let lucid patients and family members help with care plans.

Insurance

What type of insurance does the provider accept? This is one of the most important things to consider when you are searching for a company. Since most people do not have the money to pay out of pocket for all of these expenses, they will want to find a company that takes insurance to cover or offset the cost. Unfortunately, most insurance does not pay for nursing home care. Medicaid will pay, but only after you have sold your home and spent most of your money. This can be very inconvenient for your spouse. You may be able to protect your right to your home by taking a reverse mortgage, which can protect your spouse from becoming homeless after you are gone. Everyone is in a different situation, which is why you need to get a lawyer early.

Cost

How much will the service cost overall? How much will insurance cover? Get some help from family and friends when it comes to making a huge financial decision such as hiring a caregiver. Make sure that the provider will accept Medicaid if you run out of money. Many don't.

Where to Look for Providers

When you determine the type of care you need—occasional care or round-the-clock care—you can start looking for providers in your area. One of the best ways to get information on local caregivers is through your doctor. He or she will have several different choices to recommend to their patients. The doctors know these facilities better than most, and they will steer you in the right direction.

You should also contact local and national Alzheimer's disease associations. And if you know anyone who has been going through their own battle with Alzheimer's, you should talk to them or their family about the provider they use.

Personal recommendations are great, but you still need to research and verify them on your own *before* hiring. This will entail looking up the aforementioned reviews and verifying the providers' experience.

Don't forget to use the links below. The "Discovering Psychology" video series at learner.org, sponsored by The Annenberg Foundation, features very good lectures. Just click on the title on the left side of the page.

Links:

DASN International, the Dementia Advocacy and Support Network
http://www.dasninternational.org/

Annenberg Learning: "Discovering Psychology" (video series)
http://www.learner.org/series/discoveringpsychology/index.html

The Alzheimer's Association: In My Area
http://www.alz.org/apps/findus.asp

Chapter 6

Stages of Alzheimer's Disease

One of the important things to learn is that the stages of Alzheimer's are somewhat different for different people. Not all patients will experience the same symptoms at the same time. Some may never experience all of these symptoms. It depends on factors that not even doctors know right now. Still, most people will follow certain patterns or stages as the disease progresses. When you know what these seven stages are and what to expect at each one, it will make it easier for you to prepare.

Stage 1: No Impairment

At this earliest stage, there really is no difference in your cognitive function. This is the stage right before you start to notice problems with your memory and before you talk with your doctor. In fact, if a doctor were to examine you at this stage, he or she would not see any signs of dementia.

Stage 2: Very Mild Cognitive Decline

At this stage, you might have some memory lapses. You could forget where you placed your car keys or your mail. At this stage, the symptoms are still very mild, and your family, friends, and doctor will not detect any signs of dementia. In fact, you and others might chalk up your small lapses in memory to your age.

Stage 3: Mild Cognitive Decline

At this point, it *might* be possible for a doctor to diagnose Alzheimer's in an individual. However, this is not always possible. You will start to notice some more problems with your memory. Family and friends might be able to notice this as well. Some of the issues you might face at this stage include losing valuable objects, such as jewelry or wallets, forgetting material you just read, trouble in social settings, and trouble remembering names when you meet new people.

Stage 4: Moderate Cognitive Decline

At this point, the signs and the symptoms are very noticeable. You will forget events that happened very recently, and it will be very difficult to perform mathematics in your head. Making plans is more difficult, and forgetting parts of your own history becomes common. At this stage, mood and attitude often start to suffer. As your cognitive functions decline, it's natural to feel a bit moody. This is the stage I'm currently in.

Stage 5: Moderately Severe Cognitive Decline

Now there will be larger memory gaps and more significant problems with basic mental functions. During this stage you will need to start having help with your daily activities. Some of the things many patients experience at this point include confusion over place, day of the week, season, and more. Due to this, you may need to have people help you pick out clothing that's appropriate to the season. You might have even more trouble with mathematics.

Stage 6: Severe Cognitive Decline

The difficulties get worse at this stage. Some patients begin to experience personality changes. This could cause elevated suspiciousness. People will start to need more help with their daily activities. Most will still be able to remember their own name, but recent experiences leave the mind quickly, and it is difficult for patients to remember all of their personal history. Patients at this stage often need help dressing. They may forget names but they should remember most faces. Incontinence might occur, as well as delusions and hallucinations.

Stage 7: Very Severe Cognitive Decline

This is the last stage of the disease. Patients stop responding to their external environment. They lose the ability to speak and move on their own. They need to have care twenty-four hours a day.

We're All Different

Remember that these stages are the *general* way the disease progresses. You might have a different experience. Looking at the different stages and the way the disease progresses can be scary, but it should also be liberating. You know what's happening. You have the power to make the most of your time and to get your care plan in place long before you enter the latter stages of the disease.

Remember, people can live for another twenty years with Alzheimer's disease. Keep on living and making the most of each day.

Links:
The Alzheimer's Association: Seven Stages of Alzheimer's
http://www.alz.org/alzheimers_disease_stages_of_alzheimers.asp
The Alzheimer's Reading Room
http://www.alzheimersreadingroom.com/

Chapter 7

Talking with Your Family

People react differently when they learn they have Alzheimer's disease. You may be horrified, or you may be relieved. There is no typical reaction.

The first symptoms are short-term memory loss because that is the part of the brain that is damaged. You will probably be able to think clearly at first because your thinking is done in a separate part of your brain. Your brain is like a house with many rooms, each devoted to a special function. Alzheimer's is like a slow fire that makes each room unusable, but for the first years, the rest of your brain is untouched. You can still think, you can still plan, and you can still feel. In the distant future you will lose those abilities also. Everybody does—it's called death. We all die, but before that we deserve to be respected as human beings. I think it is the fear of people losing respect for us that keeps us from telling about our diagnosis.

Before you tell everyone about your Alzheimer's diagnosis, you should talk with the most trusted person in your life about it. Many people think of a dementia patient as some sort of monster. You may be better off telling them that you are having memory problems. It is a true statement, and it sounds better than "I have dementia." I tell people that I had a brain tumor (I did), but I avoid telling them that I have dementia (I do). I am at about stage 4, and I have been in this stage for over twelve years.

You can slow the progression of Alzheimer's by avoiding stress. Many people are afraid of Alzheimer's or dementia, and once you have told them you have it, you can't take it back. It will come out soon enough, so why rush it? You need time to develop your sense of humor and work on some good Alzheimer's jokes. Learn to laugh at yourself. Here's a start: Three elderly gentlemen were being tested for memory loss at the doctor's office. The doctor said, "What's three times three?" The first man said 274. The second man said Tuesday. The third man said nine. The doctor was impressed and asked the third man how he had gotten the answer. "Simple," he said. "You just subtract 274 from Tuesday." Find more at the What Makes You Laugh? Support group on Caring.com. http://www.caring.com/support-groups/caregiver-humor/31861db5

How to Tell Others

When you tell others about your disease, make sure you educate them on the subject. Just as you probably knew very little about Alzheimer's before your diagnosis, your family probably knows very little about it too. Let them know that Alzheimer's is not a normal part of aging and that it will impair your memory and your cognitive function. You might even want to go over the different stages of Alzheimer's with them so they know what to expect. You should show them AboutAlzOrg's YouTube video "What Is Alzheimer's Disease?" https://www.youtube.com/watch?v=9Wv9jrk-gXc as well. I also recommend David Shenk's book *The Forgetting: Alzheimer's: Portrait of an Epidemic.* He is a much better author than I am, but remember, I did the research to find him and others like him.

Be honest about your diagnosis. Tell your family how it makes you feel. Talk with them about how it makes *them* feel too. Even though you are the one going through the disease, it will affect their lives as well. Let their voices be heard. Answer any questions they have. If you can't answer the questions, that's fine. In fact, you probably still have quite a few questions of your own. You can consult your doctor and support groups that can help your entire family to deal with the diagnosis. Let your family know that even though the disease will cause changes to occur, you still want all of them to be a part of your life. Most of your family and your true friends will stand with you and help you when you need it. Let them know just how much you appreciate it.

Talking with Younger Children

Kids, particularly younger children, do not really grasp the concept of Alzheimer's. The KidsHealth link at the end of this chapter has some great information to help kids get a better idea of the disease and what will happen. Again, make sure that you or another family member is there to help answer all of the questions children might have.

It is important to be honest about the disease and not to sugarcoat the changes you will experience. You do not want to scare the children, but you or their parents do need to prepare them for the personality changes you may go through.

Leave Something for the Younger Generation

If you have young children or grandchildren, you may fear not being there to pass along some of your knowledge and wisdom. A good way to make sure that the children still get to benefit from your wisdom is to create a video for them. Tell them anything you want. Give them insight into life and love, or teach them how to make your best cookies or how to clean a fish.

Spend Time with Family

Right after you receive your diagnosis and tell your family, it can be a very sad time. Most people do not feel much like having fun. They wallow in their sadness. If you learn anything from this book, though, learn that your attitude makes a huge difference. Instead of feeling sad about the situation, make each day a celebration of your life. It's not time for the funeral yet—that is far in the future, maybe a lot farther than you think.

Here's another story. There were once two men who were condemned to death by the king. One begged for his life to no avail. The other, knowing the king's love for his horse, offered to teach the horse to sing. The king thought for a moment and said, "All right, I'll give you a year. If he can sing, you go free, but if he can't, you die." As they were being led away, the first convict said, "Why do you think you can teach the king's horse to sing? What a stupid idea!" The second man replied, "Well, I have a year. Maybe the king will die, maybe I'll die, and maybe the horse will sing. You, on the other hand, will be executed in the morning." The moral: stay calm, extend your time, and hope for a miracle.

Have friends over more often, take a vacation, do things with your grandkids that you've always wanted to do. Give your family great memories of you and them together. They will cherish those memories, and you will have a wonderful time. When you are happier and feeling better about life, you slow the progression of the disease.

You still have some great times left. In fact, you have more time than 95 percent of people who have a terminal illness. One thing you don't have, though, is time to waste. Get out there with all of your loved ones and enjoy those times!

Tips for Handling Memory Loss: "Where Did I Put My Keys?"

There is nothing more frustrating than losing your keys, especially when you are sure of where you left them. I try to keep mine in a jar by the front door. If I find them somewhere else, I put them in the jar. So does my wife. I also have a big colorful piece of plastic on the key ring. You have to train yourself to put your keys in the same place. Try placing a can of nuts by the jar and take one each time you put the keys there. Just do it over and over until it is automatic.

You can also buy a small cell phone and attach it to your keys. Use a felt-tip pen to write the cell number on your home phone, and write it on a card in your wallet as well. When you can't find your keys, just call the phone and it will ring, alerting you to your keys' location. Keep the phone charged and leave the charger in the same place. This works better than using one of those key-caller gadgets because you can call your keys from any phone. (Just make sure to write the number down in several places.)

To guard against locking your keys in your car, make a rule that you have to see them before you shut the door. Join AAA for those times when the keys get locked in anyway. It is nice to have a number to call for help. You do not have to be a driver to use AAA; you can call for any car that needs help.

Memory loss means losing a lot more than just keys, of course. When you lose something, first look in the places it should be, then look in places you would not expect it to be. I sometimes put my wallet in the freezer. My wife still makes jokes about "cold cash."

There will be times when you just can't find what you are looking for. You have to be able to let it go. Say, "Well, that's Alzheimer's," because that's what it is.

I use my computer for a memory aid too. It remembers to pay my bills and I use the Favorites folder to keep my place when I find something I like. I tried writing things down but soon found myself digging through piles of paper. Bottom line, do the best you can. If it doesn't work, blame it on Alzheimer's—because it is Alzheimer's.

Links:

The Alzheimer's Association: Helping Friends and Family

http://www.alz.org/living_with_alzheimers_families_and_friends.asp

KidsHealth: Grownup Conditions: Alzheimer's Disease

http://kidshealth.org/kid/grownup/conditions/alzheimers.html

Chapter 8

Treatments for Dealing with Alzheimer's and Dementia

We know there is no cure for Alzheimer's disease, but that does not mean there are no treatments that can help with some of the cognitive as well as behavioral symptoms. In this chapter, we'll cover some of the treatment options you have.

Medications

A number of medications are available for treating Alzheimer's disease. These fall into the category of cholinesterase inhibitors. According to the Alzheimer's Association, the drugs stop the breakdown of acetylcholine, a chemical messenger in the brain important for memory and learning. The drugs can delay the symptoms for between six months and a year for about 50 percent of the people who take them. There are very few side effects, though some patients do have them.

The following are some of the most popular drug options, along with possible side effects.

Aricept (Donepezil)

Aricept works at all stages of Alzheimer's disease. Some of the side effects can include nausea, vomiting, loss of appetite, and increased bowel movements. I've been taking Aricept for several years with no side effects.

Razadyne (Galantamine)

This drug is for the mild to moderate stages of Alzheimer's. The side effects exhibited by some patients are the same as those for Aricept—nausea, vomiting, loss of appetite, and increased bowel movements.

Namenda (Memantine)

Namenda works for those in the moderate to severe stages of Alzheimer's. Some of the side effects may include dizziness, confusion, constipation, and headaches.

Cognex (Tacrine)

This drug can help those in the mild to moderate stages of Alzheimer's too. The side effects can include nausea and vomiting, as well as possible liver damage.

Exelon Patch (Rivastigmine)

This patch works on mild to moderate cases. The symptoms are the same as those found in Aricept and Razadyne—nausea, vomiting, loss of appetite, and increased bowel movements.

Massage

Massage is a very effective way to treat the mental and physical effects of dementia. I am a massage therapist with special training in geriatric care. As soon as I touch someone, I can feel them relax. Blood pressure drops and anxiety is relieved. Human touch is one of the things we need to be healthy. It has no side effects and amazing benefits. See the YouTube video "The Power of Touch."
https://www.youtube.com/watch?v=PI89wM9a0Kg

Are Alternative Treatments Real?

Are there alternate treatments for Alzheimer's out there? Yes, a number of them. However, most of them are based on wishful thinking, and some are fraudulent. Wishful thinking may help; if you think something will work, it often will. Just don't spend any large sums of money on it. On the other hand, you must be very careful of fraud. There are people who will try to cheat anyone they think is impaired. Remember, anyone who tells you they can cure Alzheimer's is lying. If someone tells you that, stop talking to them and tell your doctor. The person is a criminal.

One of the issues with alternative treatments is that their effectiveness is unknown. Even worse, you do not know about the safety of the treatment. Since the

FDA does not regulate many supplements, it means you never know what you are putting into your body. In some cases, the alternative meds you try could even cause adverse reactions with prescription meds you are taking.

Before you decide to try *any* type of alternate treatments, even if it is something as seemingly mild as coral calcium, gingko biloba, or coconut oil, make sure you talk with your doctor. Everything you try is recorded in his or her notes. If you find something that works, you could help others. Your doctor can also let you know what doesn't work and protect you from scams.

In the Future

There's no cure now, but I believe there will be in the future. Doctors are working hard to find better treatments that can help to prolong your cognitive functions and life even further. Try to keep up with the changes in the field and the various options for new treatments as they come about. You might even find some clinical trials for drugs that you may wish to consider. If you are interested in a clinical trial, read Chapter 9 of P. Murali Doraiswamy's *The Alzheimer's Action Plan*. It has a very good description of what to look for and should be part of your Alzheimer's library.

Links:
The Alzheimer's Association: Treatments for Alzheimer's
http://www.alz.org/alzheimers_disease_treatments.asp
Mayo Clinic: Alzheimer's Treatments: What's on the Horizon?
http://www.mayoclinic.com/health/alzheimers-treatments/AZ00048

Chapter 9

Myth #1: Alzheimer's is a Natural Part of Aging

Alzheimer's is a disease, like cancer or heart disease. It affects older people more often than younger but is not a normal part of the aging process. Forgetting something once in a while is normal at any age. Forgetting where you live or getting lost in your own neighborhood is not. If you are worried about your memory see a doctor.

Myth #2: You Can Prevent Alzheimer's with a Healthy Lifestyle

It is important to live a healthy lifestyle. It will help you handle any disease that develops. Unfortunately it seems to have little effect on the 1 in 10 chance we all have of Alzheimer's.

I do recommend the follow "Best Practices":

1. Take meds as directed [Very Important].
2. Exercise daily—try a long walk.
3. Stretch your mind by learning something new, like playing a musical instrument [kazoos are easy] or creating art.
4. Try the Mediterranean diet.
5. Take antioxidants and omega-3 supplements.
6. Socialize, even if it is in smaller groups. Try not to lose the ability.
7. Start your morning with a smile. Think of something to look forward to.

Myth #3: Dementia and Alzheimer's are the Same Thing

Dementia is the loss of brain function and can be caused by stroke, a blow to the head, infection, or several other things.

Alzheimer's is a disease that causes dementia. It is characterized by tangles of tau protein in the neurons and plaques of beta-amyloid outside the neurons.

Myth #4: Only the Elderly Get Alzheimer's

Alzheimer's can start in your thirties. I was 48 when I was told I might have early onset Alzheimer's.

Myth #5: Treatments Stop the Progression of Alzheimer's

We have not found anything that stops the spread of Alzheimer's. I do believe that the early treatment, such as massage, drugs, and learning to laugh out loud help to slow the spread. That is why it is so important to start treatment as soon as possible. It will make a big difference in where you are in a few years.

Myth #6: Aluminum or Iron or Plastic or Aspartame or God's Curse Cause Alzheimer's

Alzheimer's is such a feared disease that people want to believe it has a cause that the can avoid. When someone comes up with a "reason" for your Alzheimer's try to understand that they are really talking to themselves. They want to believe that they can protect themselves from Alzheimer's by not doing something. The truth is that they can't, but let them have the illusion of safety. It won't help to argue with them and it will make you feel worse. Tell them you hope they will never have to face dementia and change the subject.

Myth #7: Alzheimer's is Genetic

This is not really a myth, about 10% of Alzheimer's has a genetic cause. It does not mean that all of our children will get Alzheimer's.

If you suspect your Alzheimer's was caused by genetics I advise you to tell your children to buy long term care insurance BEFORE they are tested for the Alzheimer's gene. A positive test may make it harder to buy.

Links:

The University of Bristol: “How the Human Brain Works”_(YouTube video)
http://www.youtube.com/watch?v=9UukcdU258A

AboutAlzOrg: “What Is Alzheimer's Disease?” (YouTube video)
https://www.youtube.com/watch?v=9Wv9jrk-gXc

The Alzheimer Society, Canada:_Myths and Reality about Alzheimer’s Disease
http://www.alzheimer.ca/en/About-dementia/Alzheimer-s-disease/Myth-and-reality-about-Alzheimer-s-disease

Chapter 10

Keep Living Your Life

Things are changing, and they will keep changing. It is important to make sure that you continue to live your life amid this. Once you are ready for the reality of these changes, you will find they are easier to accept. You become ready by making yourself and your environment safe and happy. In a very real way, you are going to go back to your childhood. Your body will still age but your mind will become more and more childlike.

The irony is that when you are upset, the progression of Alzheimer's happens faster. It is easy to say, "Don't get upset." The truth is that you won't be able to help it when something frustrates you. But you can avoid being upset by avoiding things that frustrate you. Losing my keys is something that really gets me. I can't leave the house without them, but that doesn't help me remember where I left them. I would run around my house, looking in the same places over and over until my wife found them for me. One day I faced my problem. I admitted that I no longer had a normal memory. The strange thing was that I never lost my keys outside my house. I realized that I always carried them in the same pocket, by habit, not choice. I did not have to remember to put them in my pocket; it was just where they always went. So I trained myself to put them in the same place in my house until it was as natural as putting them in my pocket. It worked. Now my wife might lose her keys, but I never do.

Habits are stored in a much deeper part of your brain than memory. Now is the time to develop good habits. I suggest the following: establish a normal bedtime, say ten o'clock, then a normal waking time, between six and seven o'clock. Take a bath or shower at the same time each day, clean your teeth at the same time. Think of things that cause you problems now and establish habits to help overcome them. For instance, if you can't remember instructions, carry a small notebook and pencil, and when people give you instructions, just hand over the notebook and say you have bad hearing.

Take Your Time and Plan

In the early stages, allow yourself more time to do tasks. Plan that extra time into your schedule, knowing that you won't be as fast as you once were. Trying to do things as fast as you used to will only frustrate you, and the tasks won't get done at all. Use memory aids if they help you. Some great examples include labeling drawers, keeping a list of numbers near the phone, and posting notes around the house as reminders for different tasks. These will also make your caregivers' lives much easier.

Communication

As Alzheimer's progresses, communication may become more difficult. Again, take your time when communicating. If going into social settings is difficult for you to do on your own, ask a friend or family member to accompany you. As the disease progresses, they will need to be there for you more often, but if you've spent time talking with them and preparing them, they will be ready for this.

Driving

At some point, you will no longer be able to drive. It will be too dangerous to you and to others. If you can't bear to sell your car, give your keys to someone. They can drive for you. I had to do this for several years. It is worse than it sounds, but you should do it anyway. Driving is the most dangerous thing most people do, both for themselves and for others. Think of all the accidents you have seen. Stop driving before you have one.

Keeping Your Independence as Long as Possible

There are two factors in keeping your independence, and they both depend on changing your world to allow for the changes brought about by the disease.

The first factor is mental. The second is your environment

Your house has rooms that are associated with different behaviors. You sleep in your bedroom, you cook in your kitchen, and you work in your office. But when your in-laws come to visit, you might sleep in your office and give them the bedroom. In the same way, your brain has areas that are associated with certain behaviors. When the function of one area is compromised, other areas will try to take over its function. You can help this process.

There is a part of every animal's brain that guides its actions. It does not have to think, it just knows what feels right to do. This is vital to survival and therefore resides in the deep part of his brain where it is protected from injury. We have this too. You don't have to think to walk. You don't have to think to eat. These behaviors were learned when you were an infant. You aren't aware of the signals that flow to your legs to make them move, but they have to flow to allow you to walk.

When I was a boy, I had a bad accident that cut the nerves to my right foot. I found that I could no longer walk as before. My right foot hung down and I stumbled constantly. But I could walk better if I imagined a log in my path and stepped over it. I did this until it was automatic. My brain now knows to lift my right foot higher than my left. Many years later I helped a man with Parkinson's disease to walk by telling him to "step over the log." In two weeks he could walk without stumbling. You can use this strategy too. Practice is the way to access this ability. You can replace your memory with habit. A normal person can usually remember where he put his keys. You won't, but if you have practiced enough, your keys will always be in the same place. It won't matter if you can't remember coming home; you will have made up for damage with training.

When I was a teenager, I worked in Lowery Park in Tampa. There was a man who kept trained ducks in vending machines. You put in a dime and a flag went up inside. It signaled the duck to play a piano with its beak, after which it received a treat. It was amazing. One day I asked him how long it took to train the duck. He said, "Oh, an hour or so. The secret is to start with a very hungry duck and give him one piece of food on the correct piano key. He eats it, the piano makes a note, and I put one on the next key. The hunger makes him remember where the food was and he will 'play the piano' to get more."

When you are hungry, you will remember where the food is. Try skipping a meal and putting something you like where you leave your keys. Take a bite as you put the keys down and then repeat. You will be surprised at how well you remember. There are separate “rooms” in your mind for all behaviors. They overlap and reinforce each other. When you are trying to learn something, say it out loud (speech center) as you write it down (writing center) and read it after you finish (reading center). You now have the information in four places: speech, writing, reading, and of course the written copy you made.

Try exploring your world with eyes closed. Warning—have a helper with you when you try this! Use an old fireman’s trick of putting your left hand on a wall and placing your right hand in front of you. Let sound, smell, and touch guide you. (Be careful to open your eyes when you don’t know where you are.) You don’t realize it, but vision has become the primary sense now that we have TV and computers. It is very hard to transmit smell or touch, so we have let them almost disappear. Yet they can be a tremendous help to memory. Let the world be your brain gym.

Make changes to your home to make your independence last as long as possible. The idea is to make it as safe and simple as you can. Use cues to guide your behavior. A cue is anything that reminds you to do something. For instance, a toothbrush left out can remind you to brush your teeth.

Let’s start with the outside of your home. Look for any tripping hazards and remove them if possible. If they are fixed in place, do something to make them more visible. Alzheimer’s can affect your vision and your balance.

If you plan to take walks (and you should), think about putting a cue at the end of your driveway to remind you where to turn. I use a wind chime that both moves and makes a pleasant sound to welcome me home. It also makes it much easier to give directions to my house.

You should hang something colorful on your doorknob to remind you where you live. If you live in an apartment, make it something that sticks out in the hall, like a stuffed animal, so you will remember where to go.

Keep a small table by your front door where you place your keys and other items you will need to go out. Whenever you come in, put your keys on that table. *Always place them there.* You will have to practice this, but once it becomes automatic, it will save you hours of searching.

OK, you are through your front door and you have put your keys where you can find them. Now look at your usual route in. Does it have any tripping hazards? Remove the ones you can and mark the ones you can't move. Do this throughout the house.

Your floor should be a light color with a contrasting baseboard. Avoid dark rugs—they can look like holes to Alzheimer's patients. It should be easy to see underneath your furniture (like chairs), or the furniture should be secured to the floor with boards (like beds and couches) This will save you lots of time and frustration when you are looking for dropped items.

Next it's time to remove clutter. Clutter equals confusion, and confusion will drain your energy. You will need cardboard shipping boxes, tape, and a felt-tip pen. Place everything that you don't use into the box and label it. You are not throwing anything away, just boxing it for storage. Use storage boxes because they will stack easier. Go through your whole house and repeat these steps, remove tripping hazards and boxing up clutter.

Now go to the kitchen. This can be a dangerous place, but you can make it a lot safer. Make sure you have a working smoke detector installed just outside the kitchen. Buy a fire extinguisher and mount it near the smoke detector. This is a good idea for any home. You may want to install a timer switch on your stove or at least mount a kitchen timer near it. Next check the temperature in your refrigerator. I have mine set at about thirty-three degrees. This is much colder than normal, but food keeps longer, and with dementia, you can't trust your sense of smell. Finally, label all cabinets and drawers, both for yourself and visitors. You should also get rid of any dangerous chemicals. You don't want to eat poison by mistake.

Now go in the bathroom. The big dangers here are scalds, falls, and bathroom cleaners. Set your hot water at 110 degrees. Install grab bars by your toilet and in your shower. Make sure the floor and tub have nonslip rugs or rubber mats. Replace dangerous cleaners like bleach and drain opener with hydrogen peroxide or vinegar. Leave out your toothbrush and toothpaste with a plastic cup and your hairbrush. Label any drawers and cabinets. Hang towels and put shampoo in the shower. Put in a nightlight and leave it on. Place a sign on the door so you and visitors can always find the toilet.

Now move on to the bedroom. Your bed should be comfortable and a safe distance from the floor. Place a sturdy nightstand where you can reach it from the bed. Put in a nightlight. Remove any dangerous objects. Many people keep a weapon by their bed for protection. Sorry, but it has to go. I use a plastic bottle of household ammonia for protection. If you hear someone in your home, take off the cap and hold the bottle. If they attack you, just squeeze the bottle as you aim at the chest. The ammonia makes breathing impossible and is temporarily blinding. The advantage is that it instantly renders an attacker harmless but does no permanent damage. To put it bluntly, it is a lot easier to explain why you threw ammonia on a new caregiver than why you stabbed him. I once used this method to disarm a man who had a knife.

One of the problems people face in the morning is what clothes to wear. This can be paralyzing for dementia patients. Save yourself the trouble by hanging a week's worth of outfits in your closet. Hang them in order from Monday to Sunday. You can make this into a game—it's fun, and you can let someone help you match your outfits. I recommend elastic waistbands instead of belts, as belts can be confusing. Like everything else in your life, it pays to simplify your clothing.

Finally, create a daily schedule and try to stick to it. Get up at the same time in the morning and go to bed about the same time at night. Try to shower and brush your teeth about the same time each day. As this becomes routine, it will help you with what to do next. You will develop a pattern that you can depend on to guide you on bad days.

Links:
The Alzheimer's Association: Tips for Daily Life
http://www.alz.org/living_with_alzheimers_10269.asp
ThirdAge: Living with Alzheimer's Disease
http://www.thirdage.com/hc/c/living-with-alzheimers-disease

Conclusion

There you have it. I hope you understand the main message of this book, that there is much you can do to sustain and improve your quality of life when you have Alzheimer's disease. Alzheimer's is like an infection, and the best antibiotic is laughter. It is normal to feel overwhelmed at first, but you don't have to wallow in it. I have given you several ideas to combat despair; some will work for you and some won't. The important thing is to find a way to reset your mood. We were not made to be always afraid. We were made to laugh and love and hug each moment we live, right up to the end. I hope you do.

Lose everything but your sense of humor!

John Caro

Resources

Websites

This is a list of websites and information used in the creation of this book. These links are the same ones in the chapters above. You can also click here on these links to go right to the sites you want to visit.

http://www.webmd.com/alzheimers/tc/dementia-symptoms
http://www.alz.org/living_with_alzheimers_10269.asp

http://www.mayoclinic.com/health/alzheimers/AZ00009
http://www.nia.nih.gov/alzheimers/alzheimers-disease-video

http://www.youtube.com/watch?v=7_kO6c2NfmE

http://www.alz.org/alzheimers_disease_stages_of_alzheimers.asp

http://www.alzheimersreadingroom.com/

https://www.helpforalzheimersfamilies.com/alzheimers-dementia-coping/guide/what-are-the-stages-of-alzheimers-and-dementia/

http://www.alz.org/apps/findus.asp

http://www.alz.org/living_with_alzheimers_families_and_friends.asp
http://kidshealth.org/kid/grownup/conditions/alzheimers.html
http://www.alz.org/alzheimers_disease_treatments.asp
http://www.mayoclinic.com/health/alzheimers-treatments/AZ00048

http://www.alzheimer.ca/en/About-dementia/Alzheimer-s-disease/Myth-and-reality-about-Alzheimer-s-disease

Books

I believe everybody should have an Alzheimer's library, and these books are a good start.

The 36-Hour Day: A Family Guide to Caring for People Who Have Alzheimer Disease, by Nancy L. Mace and Peter V. Rabins

The Forgetting: Alzheimer's: Portrait of an Epidemic, by David Shenk

Dancing with Rose: Finding Life in the Land of Alzheimer's, by Lauren Kessler

Still Alice, by Lisa Genova

Anatomy of an Illness: by Norman Cousins – A good book on the laughter cure.

Carved in Sand: When Attention Fails and Memory Fades in Midlife, by Cathryn Jakobson Ramin

Voices of Alzheimer's: Courage, Humor, Hope, and Love in the Face of Dementia, by Betsy Peterson

Learning to Speak Alzheimer's: A Groundbreaking Approach for Everyone Dealing with the Disease, by Joanne Koenig Coste

Losing My Mind: An Intimate Look at Life with Alzheimer's, by Thomas DeBaggio

The Alzheimer's Action Plan: What You Need to Know—and What You Can Do—About Memory Problems, from Prevention to Early Intervention and Care, by P. Murali Doraiswamy and Lisa P. Gwyther with Tina Adler

Final Exit, by Derek Humphry

If you are thinking about suicide, read this book first. It tells you what works and what doesn't. It also has a good discussion about legal issues and what happens to your loved ones. Do not attempt suicide until you read this book. The methods most people think of come from movies and do not work, but they often make your life much worse. Men usually try with a gun, women usually try with pills. Neither method works very well. A misaimed shot can blind you. An overdose of pills is almost always thrown up after you pass out and can cause massive brain damage. You can also leave your loved ones with broken hearts and bitter memories. You have plenty of time, use it wisely. I do not recommend suicide.

Other Resources

I also strongly suggest that you subscribe to Netflix. Find a comedy that makes you laugh out loud. They have films from Charlie Chaplin to modern comedy. They also carry the movie *Memento*, which I think should be seen by anyone dealing with dementia. It is hard to follow at first, but the depiction of a man who has no memory is spot on.

Don't forget YouTube, which has become the number-one place to learn anything you want to know. Just type a word into the search box. You will be amazed at what you find, and it's free.

One Last Thing

I have worked hard on this book and I would appreciate honest feedback. Please take a few minutes to leave your rating after you finish reading. Or if you would like to contact me directly, my e-mail is johncaro1@cox.net. THANK YOU

Made in the USA
Middletown, DE
09 August 2015